Sugar-Sweetened Beverage and Bone Health

Sugar-Sweetened Beverage and Bone Health

Yoo Kyoung Park
Hyejin Ahn

ELIVA PRESS

Published by Eliva Press
Email: info@elivapress.com
Website: www.elivapress.com

ISBN: 978-1-63648-247-7

Preface

Sugar-sweetened beverages (SSB), "*Sweet Temptations!*" are primary source of sugar consumption and the proportion of people consuming SSBs are steadily increasing. The health concerns of sugar-sweetened beverages are well known, such as obesity, cardiovascular disease, and dental caries. However, the effect of sugar-sweetened beverages consumption on bone health, which is difficult to confirm with the naked eye and progresses slowly, did not gain much attention.

This book comprehensively covers the effects of sugar-sweetened beverages consumption on bone mineral density, bone mineral contents and bone fracture in not only children but also adults. Most of the studies on the association between sugar-sweetened beverages and bone health published so far through systematic review of the literature were included, and through meta-analysis, we found that the consumption of sugar-sweetened beverages was associated with lower bone density.

Kyung Hee University
Republic of Korea

Yoo Kyoung Park
Hyejin Ahn

Contents

List of Figures

List of Tables

Abstract

Current evidence demonstrates that that sugar-sweetened beverages (SSBs) and bone health are related; however, there has been only a few reviews on the link between SSBs and bone health. A systematic review and meta-analysis was performed to investigate the association between SSBs consumption and bone health in children and adults. Relevant studies of SSBs and bone health published up to 15 March 2021 were searched using PubMed, the Web of Science, Cochrane Library, and a reference search. A random-effects meta-analysis was conducted to estimate the standardized mean difference (SMD). Subgroup analyses were performed to identify whether effects were modified by age, sex, measured skeletal sites, type of SSBs, and SSBs intake questionnaire. Twenty-six publications including 124,691 participants were selected on the review. The results from this meta-analysis showed a significant inverse association between SSBs intake and bone mineral density (BMD) in adults (ES: -0.66, 95% CI: -1.01, -0.31, n=4,312). Eighteen of the 20 studies included in the qualitative-only review in children and adults supported the findings from the meta-analysis. When subgroup analysis was performed according to skeletal site, a large effect was found on whole body BMD (ES: -0.97, 95% CI: -1.54, -0.40). There was a moderate effect on BMD in females (ES: -0.50, 95% CI: -0.87, -0.13). There was a moderate or large effect on BMD in individuals aged under 50 years (under 30 years: ES: -0.57, 95% CI: -0.97, -0.17; 30 to 50 years: ES: -1.33, 95% CI: -1.72, -0.93). High consumption of carbonated beverages had a moderate effect on BMD (ES: -0.73, 95% CI: -1.12, -0.35). The meta-analysis showed that SSBs consumption such as carbonated beverages were inversely related to BMD in adults. Qualitative review supported the results of meta-analysis. This review was registered in the PROSPERO database under identifier CRD 2020164428.

List of Abbreviations

ALP	alkaline phosphatase
BMC	bone mineral content
BMD	bone mineral density
BUA	broadband ultrasound attenuation
CTx	c-terminal telopeptide
DEXA	dual-energy x-ray absorptiometry
DB	distal radius
FFQ	food-frequency questionnaire
FN	femoral neck
HL	heel
HR	hazard ratio
LB	lower body
LS	lumbar spine
MR	mid-shaft radius
NTx	n-terminal telopeptide
OC	osteocalcin
pQCT	peripheral quantitative computed tomography
QUS	quantitative ultrasonography
RCT	randomized controlled trials
SEXA	single energy x-ray absorptiometry
SI	stiffness index
SMD	standardized mean difference
SOS	speed of sound
SSBs	sugar-sweetened beverages
TC	trochanter
TH	total hip
UB	upper body
USM	ultra-sonometer
WA	ward's area
WB	whole body

1. Background

Sugar-sweetened beverages (SSBs), defined as any consumable non-alcoholic water-based beverage containing significant amounts of free sugars (1), are a primary source of sugar consumption (2), and the proportion of people consuming beverages as their major source of sugar is steadily increasing (2, 3). This increase in sugar intake through beverages and its potential adverse effects on public health are of major concern (4). SSBs include non-diet soft drinks/sodas; flavored juice drinks; sports drinks; sweetened waters; coffee, tea, and milk with added sugars; energy drinks; and electrolyte replacement drinks (5). Strong evidence that SSB consumption is causally associated with increased risk of developing health problems, such as weight gain and obesity, type 2 Diabetes Mellitus, tooth decay, and cardiovascular disease, has been reported (1). Accordingly, many research and policy efforts have focused on consumption of sugar-sweetened beverages due to their substantial contribution to total added sugar intake (6, 7). The 2020 strategic Plan from the American Heart Association (AHA) recommends no more than 360 kcal per week from SSBs (8). This recommendation is exceeded by over 80% of the population in the United States (8).

Bone metabolism is affected by a variety of environmental factors, especially dietary factors (9). Given the increase in SSBs consumption over the past decade, many studies have been conducted to investigate the effect of SSBs consumption on bone health (10, 11). Added sugar, phosphoric acid, caffeine, and the acidity of SSBs may all affect bone metabolism by disturbing calcium absorption and homeostasis in the body and increasing calcium excretion through urine (12-14). High consumption of SSBs may also affect bone metabolism when replacing milk, known to be beneficial to bone health (15). Also over·consumption of SSBs is likely to accompany low diet quality (e.g. excessive intake of fast-food and low vegetable consumption), which might consequently influence micronutrient and calcium intake (16).

1

To date only one systematic review has shown a relationship between SSBs and childhood fractures (17). However, this study focused on the relationship between calcium intake and bone fracture in children, so the association between SSBs and bone fractures was not considered important. Except for this study, there are no reviews on the relationship between SSBs and bone health.

We performed a comprehensive review of the literature as well as a meta-analysis to determine the association between SSBs consumption and bone health in children and adults.

2. Materials and methods

The protocol for the systematic review and meta-analysis was registered *a priori* with the PROSPERO International Prospective Register of Systematic Reviews (CRD42020164428). PRISMA (Preferred Reporting Items for Systematic Reviews and Meta-analyses) guidelines were followed and the checklist was completed.

2-1. Data sources and searches

Systematic searches of PubMed, the Web of Science, and Cochrane Library databases for eligible studies published until the end of 15 March 2021 were performed. The search strategy is detailed in Table 1 in the Supporting Information online.

Table 1. Search strategy for a systematic review and meta-analysis assessing the association between SSB consumption and bone health in children and adults

Database	Search terms
PubMed	("carbonated drink"[Mesh] OR "fruit juice"[All Fields] OR soda[All Fields] OR "soft drink"[All Fields] OR "sports drink"[All Fields] OR "sugar-sweetened beverages"[Mesh] OR "sweetened beverage"[All Fields]) AND ("bone density"[Mesh] OR "bone fractures"[All Fields] OR "bone health"[All Fields] OR "bone mineral content"[All Fields] OR "bone mineral density"[All Fields]) *Search filter=Humans, English, Korean*
Web of Science	#1 (carbonated NEAR/3 drink*) OR (fruit NEAR/3 juic*) OR (soda*) OR (soft NEAR/3 drink*) OR (sports NEAR/3 drink*) OR (sugar NEAR/3 sweetened NEAR/3 beverag*) OR (sweetened NEAR/3 beverag*) #2 (bone NEAR/3 density) OR (bone NEAR/3 fracture*) OR (bone NEAR/3 health) OR (bone NEAR/3 mineral NEAR/3 content*) OR (bone NEAR/3 mineral NEAR/3 density) #3 #1 AND #2, *Indexes=SCI-EXPANDED, ESCI; Timespan=All years*

	#1 (carbonated NEAR/3 drink*) OR (fruit NEAR/3 juic*) OR (soda*) OR (soft NEAR/3 drink*) OR (sports NEAR/3 drink*) OR (sugar NEAR/3 sweetened NEAR/3 beverag*) OR (sweetened NEAR/3 beverag*)
Cochrane Library	#2 (bone NEAR/3 density) OR (bone NEAR/3 fracture*) OR (bone NEAR/3 health) OR (bone NEAR/3 mineral NEAR/3 content*) OR (bone NEAR/3 mineral NEAR/3 density)
	#3 #1 AND #2, *Search filter= All Text*

Studies that investigated the association between SSBs consumption and bone health written in English and Korean were included. If the title, abstract, and keywords seemed relevant, the full-text of the record was assessed. Abstract, reviews and meta-analyses, studies with no relevant data, studies with non-relevant exposure or non-relevant outcomes, and duplicates were excluded. In addition, we performed manual searches of reference lists of relevant reviews and articles included in the systematic review. The literature search was performed without restrictions on study design or publication date. Ethical approval was not required for the present study. Further details of the search strategy are provided in Figure 1.

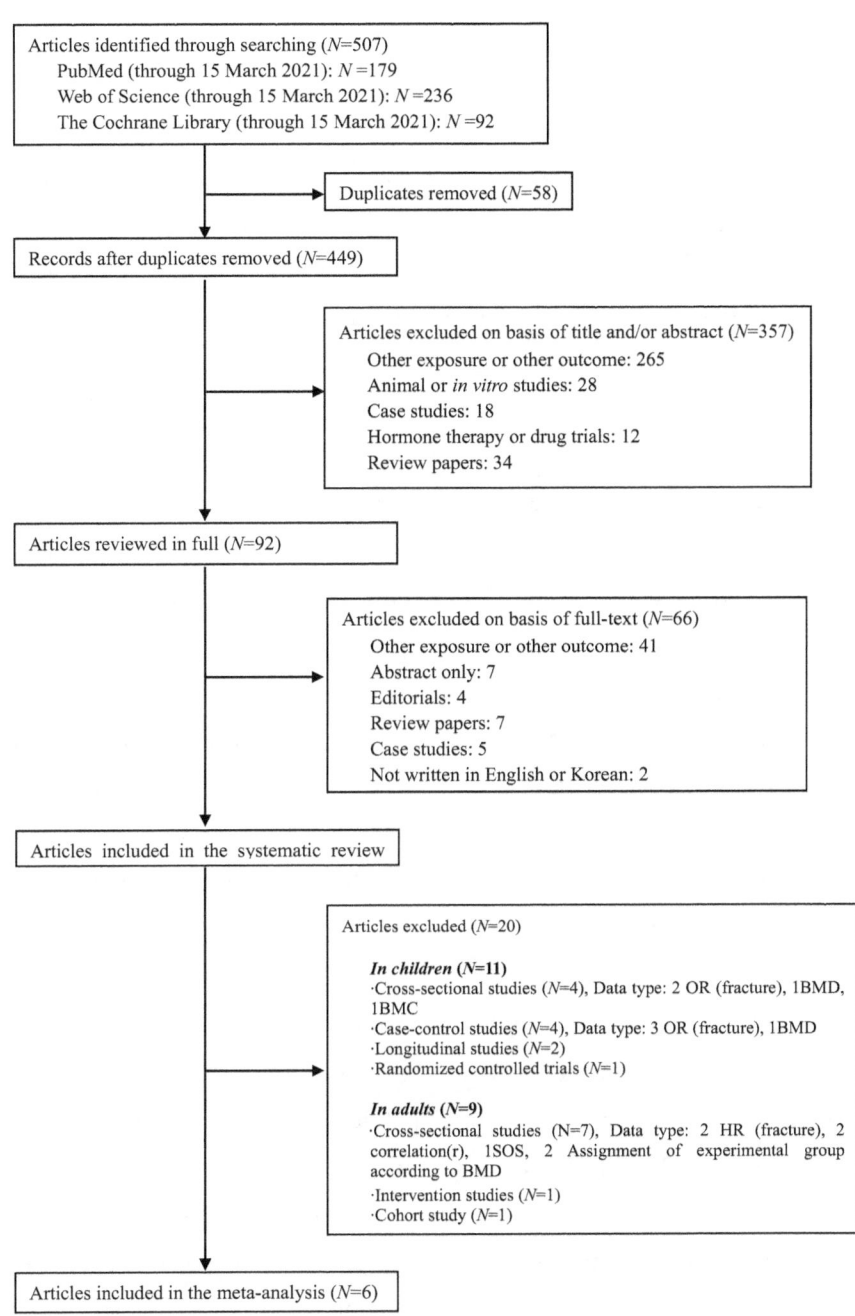

Figure 1. Flowchart of literature search and selection of studies.

2-2. Study selection

The following criteria were applied to identify articles for inclusion in our systematic review and meta-analysis: 1) studies involving healthy people without coexisting medical conditions or treatments affecting bone metabolism; 2) studies presenting a relationship between SSBs consumption and bone-related parameters [bone mineral content (BMC), bone mineral density (BMD), or bone fractures]; and 3) studies reporting levels of bone-related parameters for groups with different consumption of SSBs. No study design or time restrictions were applied when searching the databases. Among the studies included in the systematic review, the criteria applied to the studies in the meta-analysis are as follows: 1) comparative studies of groups who consumed more than 1cup or less of SSBs per day; 2) studies presenting a relationship between SSBs consumption and BMD; 3) cross-sectional studies. We excluded studies with no comparative group, reviews, editorials, and in *vivo/vitro* studies.

Two investigators (H.A. and YKP.) independently screened the titles, abstracts, and keywords of the articles to evaluate eligibility for inclusion. If consensus was reached, articles were either excluded or a full text of the study was retrieved. Full texts of the selected articles were appraised critically to determine eligibility for inclusion in the review. Disagreements were resolved by discussion between the investigators until consensus was reached.

2-3. Data extraction and quality assessment

All data were extracted by HA and checked by YKP. Extracted data included: 1) publication characteristics (author, publication year, geographic location, and sample size); 2) population (total number of participants, health status, age, sex ratio); 3) study design (intervention study, case-control study, or cross-sectional study); 4) exposure (assessment method and type of SSBs intake); 5) outcome (assessment method and bone-related parameters); 6) confounders (factors that analyses were adjusted for or matched on). If bone-related parameters were reported

6

in different units to the most commonly used units, data were converted. When necessary, we contacted the authors of the primary studies to obtain additional information. Means and SDs were calculated for BMD or BMC and risk estimates were expressed as ORs, RRs or HRs with corresponding 95% CIs.

Two investigators (H.A. and Y.K.P.) independently evaluated the quality of cohort studies and case-control studies using the Newcastle–Ottawa quality assessment scale (18, 19) for the following criteria: representativeness and selection; comparability; assessment of outcome or exposure, which ranges 0~9 (good quality for ≥7, fair quality for ≥5). The quality of the intervention study was assessed using validated checklists published by the National Institutes of Health (20) ranging 0~14 (good quality for ≥11, fair quality for ≥8). The quality of cross-sectional (observational) studies was evaluated using Handel's scale (17) for the reporting of observational studies in the field of nutrition. This quality assessment includes five quality categories: selection of study participants, measurement of outcome variables, description of withdrawals or dropouts, control for confounding bias, and application of an adequate statistic. Ten questions were given a grade based on a 5-point scale, and studies with scores of more than half of the total score were evaluated for good quality and fairness.

2-4. Statistical analysis

BMD is usually expressed in g/cm^2, and rarely as Z scores or T scores. To allow pooling of data, BMD values from each study were converted into a treatment effect size (ES) with its 95% CI, in accordance with the Hedges method, which is designed for quantitative data (21).

Statistical analyses were performed using the R program (mate-package, version 3.6.3). We conducted a meta-analysis according to a random-effects model (Hedge's method) for the main effect outcomes by combining inverse variance-weighted study-specific estimates (22). We calculated standardized mean difference (SMD) between two groups for measuring ES, which is used as a summary statistic in most of the meta-analysis when the studies all uses similar outcome measures, but, measured with various methods. Forest plots were used to visualize individual and summarize estimates, and the Cochrane Q statistic and I^2 statistic calculated using the formula [(Q-df)/Q]x100% were used to evaluate between-study heterogeneity (23, 24). We considered an effect size of 0.30 or less to be "small", an effect size of 0.40 to 0.70 to be "medium", and an effect size of 0.80 or above to be "large" (25). An I^2 value >50% was generally considered to be high (26). Subgroup analysis to explore heterogeneity was performed with pre-specified potential confounders such as age, sex, measured skeletal sites, type of SSBs, and SSBs intake questionnaire (27, 28).

3. Results

3-1. Literature search and selection

We screened 507 references and confirmed 449 references as potential studies for review after removal of duplicates. Articles were excluded on the basis of title and/or abstract (n=357), and then excluded on the basis of full text (n=66). Finally, we included 26 references (29-54) involving 124,691 participants in this systematic review (n=20) and meta-analysis (n=6). Twenty studies were excluded from our meta-analysis, as the number of studies in which the study design and bone-related indicators matched was small. Excluded studies were reviewed qualitatively. Finally, the association between SSBs and BMD was assessed based on six references involving 4,312 participants. The list of excluded reasons for exclusion are given in Figure 1.

3-2. Study characteristics

The characteristics of studies included in this systematic review and meta-analysis are summarized in Tables 2 and 3. Original articles in this review were published over the period from 1997-2020. The 26 studies included in the review were from the United States of America (n=8), South Korea (n=4), Egypt (n=1), England (n=2), Saudi Arabia (n=2), Australia (n=1), Canada (n=1), Chile (n=1), China (n=1), Denmark (n=1), Germany (n=1), Greece (n=1), New zealand (n=1) and Norway (n=1), with individuals aged from 4 to 98 years. The number of participants in these 26 studies totaled 124,691 and ranged from 98 to 73,572.

Individual SSBs evaluated were carbonated/soda/soft beverages in 21 studies, sugar-sweetened beverages in four studies, and coffee with sugar or syrup in one study. The studies used a variety of methods to assess the amount of SSBs intake including food-frequency questionnaires (FFQs) or modified FFQs (n=11), 24-hr recall (n=2), 3-day food record (n=3), diet history (n=1), and questionnaires developed by the authors (n=8).

BMD and other bone-related parameters were measured by dual-energy X-ray absorptiometry (DEXA, n=11), ultra-sonometry (USM, n=3), quantitative ultrasonography (QUS, n=3), peripheral quantitative computed tomography (pQCT, n=1), or single energy x-ray absorptiometry (SEXA, n=1) at the distal radius (DR), femoral neck (FN), forearm, heel, lower body (LB), lumbar spine (LS), mid-shaft radius (MR), whole body (WB), whole femur (WF), total hip (TH), trochanter (TC), and/or Ward's area (WA).

3-3. Qualitative review of studies not included in the meta-analysis

Association between SSBs consumption on bone health in children

The relationship between SSBs consumption and bone health in children and adolescents was investigated in eight articles (Table 2). Of these, six studies (30, 31, 33-36) reported a significantly inverse relationship between SSBs intake and bone health (two longitudinal studies, three cross sectional studies, and one case-control study). Two longitudinal studies (30, 31) performed over a 4-year period found a significant inverse relationship between SSBs consumption and forearm BMC ($p=0.036$) or whole-body BMD ($p<0.001$) in children and adolescents. Three cross-sectional studies (33, 34, 36) also reported a significant inverse relation between SSBs intake and BMC (Manias: spine: $p=0.001$; upper body, $p<0.0001$; lower body, $p=0.001$; Whiting: carbonated drinks, $p=0.05$; low nutrient dense beverages, $p=0.03$), BMD (Manias: spine: $p=0.0003$; upper body, $p=0.015$; lower body, $p=0.015$; McGartland: forearm, $p<0.05$; heel, $p<0.05$), or speed of sound (SOS; forearm, $p=0.002$). Of these, two studies in particular (34, 36) reported significant inverse relationships between SSBs consumption and bone health in girls only. One case-control study (35) presented inverse relation between SSBs consumption and BMD ($p<0.001$) in children. The eight articles involving children and adolescents that studied the link between SSBs consumption and bone health had inconsistent study designs and bone-related parameters. Therefore, we could not conduct a meta-analysis of these studies.

Table 2. Characteristics of the eight observational studies on associations between sugar-sweetened beverage consumption and bone health in children[1,2]

First author years (Ref) location	Study design	Sample size	Age range (y)	Sugar-sweetened beverages			Bone health			
				Method of assessment	Beverage category	Intake level	Method of assessment	Sites	Outcomes	Main finding
Albala 2008(29)[3] Chile	Randomized controlled trial	98	8–10	Modified FFQ	Sugar-sweetened beverages[4]	Low: 742.8±207.9[5] High: 802.1±142.0 p=0.10 g/d	DEXA	WB	Bone Mass	·No difference in whole body bone mass between children fed different amounts of sugar-sweetened beverages (p=0.56).
Fisher 2004(30)[3] USA	Longitudinal study	182	9	24-hr dietary recall	Sweetened beverages[6]	Low: 358 High: 403, g/d	DEXA	WB	BMD	·Girls who drank more sweetened beverages (p<0.01) had a significantly lower whole-body BMD (p<0.001).
Libuda 2008(31) Germany	Longitudinal study	228	6–18	3-day food records	Soft drinks	*8y, Prepubescent* Girls: 119.8±129.2 Boys: 136.8±137.3 *13y, Pubescent* Girls: 186.0±196.5 Boys: 243.5±200.4, g/d	pQCT	Forearm	BMC	·Soft drinks consumption in children and adolescents was inversely associated with BMC at forearm (p=0.036).
Ma 2004(32) Australia	Case-control study	390	9–16	Questionnaire developed by author	Carbonated or cola drinks	Not reported	DEXA	WB LS FN	BMD	·No significant correlation was shown between carbonated and/or cola drinks and bone measures, although all were inverse trends.
Manias 2006(33) England	Case-control study	100	4–16	FFQ	Carbonated beverages	Low: 0.13±0.17 High: 0.33±0.57 p=0.0182, ℓ/d	DEXA	LS UB LB	BMD BMC	·Children who consumed more carbonated drinks (p=0.0182) had a significantly lower BMD and BMC z-score at spine (BMD, p=0.0003; BMC, p=0.001), upper body (BMD, p=0.015; BMC, p<0.0001) and lower body (BMD, p=0.015; BMC, p=0.001).

11

Reference	Study type	N	Method	Dietary exposure	Intake			Outcome	Results
McGartland 2003 (34) England	Cross-sectional study	1335	12–15	Dietary history	Carbonated soft drinks[7]	12y: Girls: 351±332 Boys: 459±394, $p<0.01$ 15y: Girls: 340±380 Boys: 518±452, $p<0.01$, g/d	DEXA	DR HL	BMD	·A significant inverse relationship between total intake of carbonated soft drinks and BMD was observed in girls at the forearm ($p<0.05$) and heel ($p<0.05$).

Table 2: (*Continued*)

First author years (Ref) location	Study design	Sample size	Age range (y)	Sugar-sweetened beverages			Bone health			Main finding
				Method of assessment	Beverage category	Intake level	Method of assessment	Sites	Outcomes	
Nassar 2014 (35) Eqypt	Case-control study	100	Low: 10.3±1.4 High: 10.6±1.3	Questionnaire developed by author	Sugar-sweetened beverages[4]	Low: 1.08±0.64 *High*: 3.16±0.37 $p<0.001$ number of intake /day[8]	DEXA	LS	BMD	·Children who consumed more than 12 ounces had a significantly lower BMD ($p<0.001$) than those that does not exceed 0-8 ounces.
Whiting 2001 (36) Canada	Cross-sectional study	112	10-16 y	24-hr recall	Carbonated and low nutrient-density beverages[9]	*Girls* ·Carbonated, 96±102 ·Low nutrient dense, 240±177 *Boys* ·Carbonated, 246±300 ·Low nutrient density, 429±393 mL/d	DEXA	WB	BMC	·Consumption of carbonated ($p=0.05$) and low nutrient dense beverages ($p=0.03$) was inversely related to BMC in adolescent girls but not in boys.

[1]BMC, bone mineral content; BMD, bone mineral density; d, day; DEXA, Dual-energy X-ray absorptiometry; DR, Distal radius; F, Female; FFQ, Food frequency questionnaire; FN, Femoral neck; High, high intake of SSBs; HL, Heel; LB, Lower body; Low, low intake of SSBs; LS, Lumbar spine; pQCT, peripheral quantitative computed tomography; QUS, Quantitative ultrasonography; Ref, Reference; SD, Standard deviation; SOS, speed of sound; WB, Whole body; UB, Upper body; USA, United States of America; y, year.

[2]Quality assessment was performed using the Cochrane criteria and Handel's-developed scale and assessed by two authors (HA and YKP).

[3]Standard errors (SE) presented in the original articles were converted to standard deviations (SD) for meta-analysis. This formula was used for conversion: SD=SE X √n.

[4]'*Sugar-sweetened beverage*' included carbonated beverages and juice drinks-made by adding packaged sugary powders with fruit flavoring to water

[5]Values are means ± SD (all such values).

[6]'*Sweetened Beverage*' included both energy-containing carbonated (soda) and noncarbonated beverages (fruit drinks, sport drinks, sweetened iced tea) that contained little if any fruit juice

[7]'*Carbonated soft drinks*' were defined as all nonalcoholic carbonated beverages that contained artificial sweeteners instead of added sugar.

[8]First, children with a daily intake of more than 12 ounces of SSBs or less than 0-8 ounces of SSBs were recruited. After that, the number of drinks they consumed per day was investigated.

[9]'*Carbonated beverages*' includes cola, diet cola and other soft drinks; and '*low nutrient dense beverages*' is the sum of carbonated and noncarbonated beverages. The latter included sugared drinks such as iced tea, Koolaid, coffee<50% fruit juice, and fruit punches.

13

Association between SSBs consumption on bone health in adults

The association between SSBs consumption and bone health in adults was investigated in twelve articles (Table 3). All six articles (40, 41, 44, 46-47) excluded from the meta-analysis reported significant inverse associations between SSBs consumption and bone health in adults (five cross-sectional studies and one interventional study). Hostmark et al. (40) found a inverse association between SSBs intake and forearm BMD (cola, $p=0.012$; non-cola soft drinks, $p=0.026$). Supple et al. (46) reported an inverse association between SSBs consumption and heel BMD ($p<0.0001$). Meanwhile, Tucker et al. (47) found a inverse association between SSBs intake and BMD in women (TH, $p<0.01$; TC, $p<0.01$; FN, $p<0.001$; WA, $p<0.001$) but not in men. Kristensen et al. (44) reported that SSBs consumption (cola 2.5 L/day) for 10 days increased bone turnover.

Association between SSBs consumption on bone fracture

Eight articles (32, 33, 49-54) examined the association between SSBs intake and bone fractures (Table 4). Three studies (49, 50, 52) reported the SSBs consumption was associated with an elevated HR or OR of bone fractures in adults (Chen: HR 4.69, 2.80, 7.88; Fung: RR 1.42, 1.15, 1.74; Kremer: HR 1.26, 1.01, 1.56). Four artivles (32, 50, 53, 54) found that excessive SSBs intake was associated with a higher bone fracture risk in children and adolescent (Delshed: Boy OR 2.0, 1.0, 4.3; Delshed: Girls OR 4.6, 2.3, 9.1; Ma: OR 1.39, 95% CI: 1.01, 1.91, $p<0.05$; Petridou: cola OR 1.7, 95% CI: 1.2, 2.6, $p=0.007$, non-carbonated beverages OR 1.6, 95% CI: 1.1, 2.3, $p=0.017$; Wyshak: carbonated beverages OR 3.14, 95% CI: 1.45, 6.78, $p=0.004$, colas OR 2.01, 95% CI: 1.17, 3.43, $p=0.011$). The other case-control study (33) reported that SSBs intake was higher in the fracture group than the non-fracture group (fracture group: 0.25±0.44 L/d; non-fracture group: 0.13±0.17 L/d; $p=0.0161$).

14

Table 3. Characteristics of the twelve observational studies on associations between sugar-sweetened beverages consumption and bone health in adults[1,2]

First author, years (Ref), location	Study design	Sample size	Age range (y)	Sugar-sweetened beverage consumption			Bone health			Main finding
				Method of assessment	Types	Intake levels or categories	Method of assessment	Sites	Outcomes	
Alghadir,2015 (37) Saudi Arabia Young, M Young, W Old, M Old, W	Cross-sectional study	100 86 60 104	25–30 31–45	Questionnaire developed by author[3]	Carbonated Beverage	Low: Normal[4,5] (<3 cups/wk) High: High (≥3 cups/wk)	DEXA	WB	BMD	·Men and women in both younger and older groups who consumed more than 3 cups of carbonated beverages per day had a significantly lower whole-body BMD than did those who consumed less than 3 cups (young, M, p<0.01; young, W, p<0.01; old, M, p<0.01; old, W, p<0.01)
Cho 2008 (38) South Korea	Cross-sectional study	229	18–29	Questionnaire developed by author[6]	Carbonated Beverage	Low: Not at all High: Often (≥1 serving per day)	USM	HL	BMD SOS	·No difference in heel BMD T-score between women who often consumed carbonated beverages and who did not consume carbonated beverages (p=0.07). However, SOS levels of women who often consumed carbonated beverages was lower than those of women who did not consume carbonated beverages (p=0.03).
Hammad 2017 (39) Saudi Arabia	Cross-sectional study	101	20–24.9	Modified FFQ[7]	Soft drinks	Low: Rare (<1 can/d) High: Frequent (>3 cans/d)	QUS	HL	BMD SI	·Participants with frequent consumption of soft drinks had significantly lower T-scores and Z-scores for heel BMD than those with rare soft drink intake (Z-score, p=0.02; T-score, p=0.02). ·Soft drink intake was inversely associated with T-score and Z-score of BMD and SI at the heel (T-score, p=0.003; Z-score, p=0.002; SI, p=0.02).
Hostmark 2011 (40) Norway	Cross-sectional study	2,126	30–60	FFQ	Soft drinks	Not reported	SEXA	DR	BMD	·Cola and non-cola soft drink consumption was inversely associated with distal forearm BMD (cola, p=0.012; non-cola soft drinks, p=0.026), whereas consumption of fruit juice was not associated with distal forearm BMD when covariates were adjusted for.
Jeong 2010 (41) South Korea	Cross-sectional study	160	about 20	Modified FFQ[8]	Carbonated Beverage	Low: 51.3±74.6 High: 92.9±114.1 g/d, p<0.05	USM	HL	BMD BUA SI	·Women who consumed more carbonated beverages (p<0.05) had significantly lower T-score (p<0.001) and Z-score (p<0.001) heel BMD and showed significantly lower SI (p<0.001) and BUA(p<0.001).
Kim 1997 (42)[9] USA	Cross-sectional study	1,000	44–98	Questionnaire developed by author	Carbonated Beverage	Low: Nondrinkers or occasional drinkers High: Drinkers (≥1 serving./d)	DEXA	LS, TH DR, MR	BMD	·No difference in BMD at the distal radius, mid-shaft radius, total hip, or lumbar spine was observed between women who drank or did not drink/ occasionally drank carbonated beverages.

Table 3. *(Continued)*

(Continued)

First author, years (Ref), location	Study design	Sample size	Age range(y)	Sugar-sweetened beverage consumption			Bone health			Main finding
				Method of assessment	Types	Intake levels or categories	Method of assessment	Sites	Outcomes	
Kim 2020 (43) South Korea	Cross-sectional study	2,499	12-25	Dietary records	Cola	Low: Non-cola drinker High: Cola drinker	DEXA	WB, WF FN, LS	BMD	· No difference in BMD at the whole body, whole femur, femoral neck, and lumbar spine was observed between participants who drank or did not drink carbonated beverage.
Kristensen 2005 (44) Denmark	Intervention study	11	22-29	-	Cola	2.5 L/d during 10 days	-	Serum	OC, ALP CTx, NTx	· High consumption of cola over a 10-day period with a low-calcium diet reduced serum levels of OC. High intake of cola increased bone turnover compared to high intake of milk.
Pettinato 2006 (45) USA	Cross-sectional study	151	11–26	Modified FFQ	Soda	Girls: 2.1 ± 3.1 Boys: 1.1 ± 1.5 $p=0.012$, cups/d	QUS	DR	SOS	· Inverse correlation found between non-diet soda and the radical SOS at forearm in girls ($p=0.002$), but not in boys.
Supplee 2011 (46) USA	Cross-sectional study	438	>18	FFQ	Soda	1.7 servings/d	QUS	HL	BMD	· Soda consumption in the unadjusted model was positively and significantly associated with BMD ($p<0.0001$). In the fully-adjusted model, however, soda consumption was no longer associated with BMD.
Tucker 2006 (47) USA	Cross-sectional study	2,538	30–87	FFQ	Soft drinks	Not reported	DEXA	TH, TC FN, WA	BMD	· Soft drink intake was associated with significantly lower BMD at each hip site (TH, $p<0.01$; TC, $p<0.01$; FN, $p<0.001$; WA, $p<0.001$) in women but not in men.
Yeon 2009 (48) South Korea	Cross-sectional study	133	18–23	Dietary records	Coffee with syrup or sugar	Low:95.8 ± 163.5 High:194.5 ± 168.6, $p<0.05$, g/d	USM	HL	BMD	· No difference was observed in heel BMD between groups that consumed different amounts of beverages and coffee with sugar/syrup.

[1]ALP, alkaline phosphatase; BMD, bone mineral density; BUA, broadband ultrasound attenuation; CTx, c-terminal telopeptide; d, day; DEXA, dual-energy x-ray absorptiometry; DR, distal radius; F, female; FFQ, food frequency questionnaire; FN, femoral neck; High, high intake of SSBs; HL, heel; Low, low intake of SSBs; LS, lumbar spine; MR, mid-shaft radius; NTx, n-terminal telopeptide; OC, osteocalcin; QUS, quantitative ultrasound; Ref, reference; SD, standard deviation; SEXA, single energy x-ray absorptiometry; SI, stiffness index; SOS, speed of sound; WB, whole body; WF, whole femur; TC, trochanter; TH, total hip; USA, United States of America; USM, ultra-sonometer; WA, ward's area; wk, week. [2]Quality assessment was performed using the Cochrane criteria and Handel's-developed scale and assessed by two authors (HA and YKP). [3] Beverage consumption was subdivided into subcategories: i. Tea or coffee (caffeine-containing beverages), ii. Alcoholic beverages (alcohol, beer or wine), iii. Carbonated sugary beverages (such as cola beverages) or other soft drinks, iv. Milk intake. [4]Values are means ± SD (all such values). [5]Participants with soft drink intake were divided into normal (less than average) and high groups (equal or more than average). [6]The tool for lifestyle measurement consisted of 14 items known to be directly related to bone mineral density, including carbonated beverages. [7]A simple food-frequency questionnaire was used, indicating the number of times per week that these foods were eaten and whether the portion size was large in the case of soft drinks. [8]Based on Korean National Nutrition Survey 2008; frequently consumed food items based on amount and frequency were selected. [9]95% confidence interval (CI) presented in this original article was converted to standard deviation (SD) for meta-analysis using the following formula: SD=(Mean–Lower endpoint/1.96) X √n or SD=(Upper endpoint-Mean/1.96) X √n

16

Table 4. Characteristics of the eight studies on the effect of sugar-sweetened beverage consumption on bone fractures in children and adults[1,2]

First author year (Ref) location	Study design	Sample size	Age range	Main finding[3]
Chen 2020 (49) China	Cross-sectional and longitudinal study	9,914	20-75 y	**Frequency of soft drinks consuption** · 1-2times/wk: HR 1.17 (0.81, 1.67) · 3-4times/wk: HR 1.13 (0.58, 2.21) · Almost Daily: HR 4.69 (2.80, 7.88) **Soft drinks consuption** · <1L/wk: HR 0.96 (0.75, 1.24) · ≥1L/wk: HR 1.16 (0.83, 1.61)
Delshad 2020 (50) New Zealand	Cross-sectional study	647	8-12 y	·Boy OR 2.0 (1.0, 4.3)[4] ·Girls OR 4.6 (2.3, 9.1)[4]
Fung 2014 (51) USA	Cohort study	73,572	50 y and older (postmenopausal women)	**Total soda** RR 1.42 (1.15, 1.74), p=0.0004***[5] RR 1.14 (1.06, 1.23) per daily serving[6] **Regular soda** RR 1.37 (0.90, 2.10), p=0.03* RR 1.19 (1.02, 1.38) per daily serving **Diet soda** RR 1.38 (1.06, 1.81), p=0.007** RR 1.12 (1.03, 1.21) per daily serving **Caffeinated soda** RR 1.18 (0.82, 1.70), p=0.02* RR 1.15 (1.02, 1.29) per daily serving **Non-caffeinated soda** RR 1.56 (1.16, 2.09), p=0.19 RR 1.08 (0.97, 1.20) per daily serving **Cola** RR 1.18 (0.81, 1.71), p=0.07 RR 1.12 (0.99, 1.26) per daily serving **Non-cola** RR 1.25 (0.87, 1.79), p=0.007** RR 1.32 (1.08, 1.62) per daily serving
Kremer 2019 (52) USA	Cross-sectional and cohort study	27,617	50-79 y (postmenopausal women)	**Total soda** ·Up to 2 serving/wk: HR 1.03 (0.93, 1.13) ·2.1-5 serving/wk: HR 1.00 (0.88, 1.14) ·5.1-14 serving/wk: HR 1.07 (0.94, 1.23) ·>14 serving/wk: HR 1.26(1.01, 1.56)

(Continued)

Table 4. (*Continued*)

First author year (Ref) location	Study design	Sample size	Age range	Main finding[3]
Ma 2004 (32) Australia	Case-control study	390	9-16 y	**Cola drink** ·Hand OR 1.41 (0.71, 2.82) ·Wrist and forearm OR 1.39 (1.01, 1.91), p<0.05* ·Upper arm OR 0.65 (0.36, 1.17) **Carbonated drink** ·Hand OR 1.11 (0.71, 1.74) ·Wrist and forearm OR 1.14 (0.89, 1.46) ·Upper arm OR 1.00 (0.63, 1.58)
Manias 2006 (33) England	Case-control study	100	4-16 y	·SSBs intake(L/day) ·Non-fracture groups: 0.13±0.17 ·Fracture group: 0.25±0.44, p=0.0161*[7] -One fracture: 0.16±0.19, p=0.07163[7] -Recurrent fractures: 0.33±0.57, p=0.0182*[6], p=0.0359*[8]
Petridou 1997 (53) Greece	Case-control study	200	7-14y	·Carbonated non-cola beverages: OR 1.1 (0.7, 1.8), p=0.641 ·Cola beverages: OR 1.7 (1.2, 2.6), p=0.007** ·Non-carbonated beverages: OR 1.6 (1.1, 2.3), p=0.017*
Wyshak 2000 (54) USA	Cross-sectional study	460	14-16y	·Carbonated beverages: OR 3.14 (1.45, 6.78), p=0.004** ·Colas: OR 2.01 (1.17, 3.43), p=0.011*

[1]*p<0.05, **p<0.01, ***p<0.001. 95% CI, 95% confidence interval; d, day; F, female; HR, Hazard ratio; OR, odd ratio; Ref, reference; RR, risk ratio; SD, standard deviation; SSBs, sugar-sweetened beverages; wk, week; y, year.
[2]Quality assessment was performed using the Newcastle-Ottawa scale and Handel's-developed scale and assessed by two authors (HA and YKP).
[3]Values are mean±SD, ORs (95% CIs), RRs (95% CIs) or HRs (95% CIs).
[4]ORs for SSBs drinks and bone fractures when men and women who consumed ≥1 serving/d were compared with those consumed <1 serving/d.
[5]RRs for SSBs drinks and hip fractures when women who consumed ≥10 serving/wk were compared with non-consumers.
[6]RRs per serving per day (12 fluid ounces, 355 ml)
[7]p values refer to the significance of results compared to the non-fracture group (t-test).
[8]P values refer to the significance of results compared to the one fracture group (t-test).

3-4. Quantitative review of associations between SSBs consumption and BMD in adults; *A meta-analysis*

The relationship between SSBs consumption and BMD in men and women is presented in Figure 2, and individual effect sizes are shown in Table 5. This analysis was based on six studies including 4,312 adults. We found a significant inverse association between SSBs consumption and BMD in adults (ES: -0.66, 95% CI: -1.01, -0.31; I^2: 91%; quantifying heterogeneity test, $p<0.01$). Among the six studies of adults, two studies (37, 39) found a significant inverse association between SSBs consumption and BMD. Meanwhile, the other four studies (42, 48) found no significant association. Alghadir et al. (37) reported a significantly lower whole-body BMD in all four participant groups (young men, young women, older men, and older women) who drank ≥3 cups SSBs/week than in those who drank <3 cups SSBs/week (SSBs, $p<0.01$; BMD, $p<0.01$). Hammad et al. (39) also reported that participants with frequent consumption of soft drinks (>3 cans/day) showed significantly lower heel BMD T-scores and Z-scores that those with rare soft drink intake (<1 can/day) (Z-score, $p=0.02$; T-score, $p=0.02$). Meanwhile, Cho et al. (38), Kim et al. (42) and Kim et al. (43) found no significant association between SSBs and BMD between participants who drank ≥1 serving/day and non-/occasional drinkers or between participants who drank SSBs 'often' or 'not at all.' Yeon et al. (48) also found no significant association between SSBs and BMD when comparing women who consumed an average of 194.5 g/day of SSBs and those who consumed an average of 95.8 g/day, even though the SSBs consumption of the two groups differed significantly ($p<0.05$).

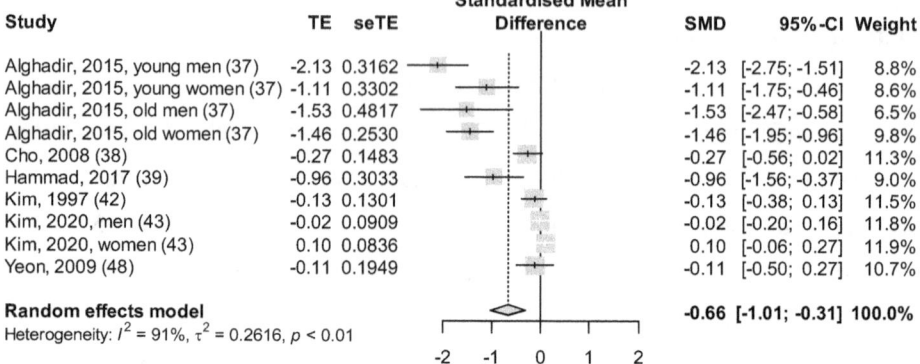

Figure 2. Forest plot of association between sugar-sweetened beverage consumption and bone mineral density in adults

Statistical analyses were performed using the R program (mate-package, version 3.6.3). We conducted a meta-analysis according to a random-effects model (Hedge's method) for the main effect outcomes by combining inverse variance-weighted study-specific estimates. Squares and horizontal lines represent the effect size and 95% CI for individual studies, and the area of each square is proportional to the study's weight in the meta-analysis. Diamond and dashed vertical lines represent the overall effect size and 95% CI in the meta-analysis. The I^2 and P values for heterogeneity are shown. SMD, standardized mean difference; 95% CI, 95% confidence interval; W, weight.

Table 5. Individual effect sizes from studies included in the meta-analysis[1.]

First author	Sites assessed	No. assessed	Effect size (g)	Variance (g)
Alghadir, 2015(37), Young man	Whole body	100	-2.128†	0.100
Alghadir, 2015(37), Young women	Whole body	86	-1.103†	0.109
Alghadir, 2015(37), Old man	Whole body	60	-1.526†	0.232
Alghadir, 2015(37), Old women	Whole body	104	-1.455†	0.064
Cho, 2008 (38)	Heel	229	-0.270	0.022
Hammad, 2017 (39)	Heel	101	-0.962†	0.092
Kim, 1997 (42)	Total hip		0.064	0.017
	Lumbar spine	1,000	0.000	0.017
	Ultra-distal radius		-0.192	0.017
	Mid-shaft radius		-0.230	0.017
Kim, 2020 (43), Man	Whole femur		-0.062	0.008
	Femoral neck	1,222	-0.024	0.008
	Lumbar spine		-0.030	0.008
	Heel		0.026	0.008
Kim, 2020 (43), Woman	Whole femur		0.000	0.007
	Femoral neck	1,277	0.080	0.007
	Lumbar spine		0.151	0.007
	Heel		0.156	0.007
Yeon, 2009 (48)	Heel	105	-0.114	0.038

[1]ES, effect size; 95% CI, 95% confidence interval. ES of 0.30 or less is regarded as small, 0.40 to 0.70 as medium, and 0.80 or above as large (24). †Effect size is significant with 95% CI.

3-5. *Qu*antitative review of associations between SSBs consumption and BMD in adults; *A meta-analysis (Subgroup analysis)*

There was a significant inverse association between SSBs and BMD in adults (random-effects models, ES: -0.66, 95% CI: -1.01, -0.31) and significant heterogeneity (I^2=91%; quantifying heterogeneity test, p<0.01). We therefore conducted subgroup analyses according to age, sex, measured skeletal site and type of SSBs, and SSBs intake questionnaire.

Individual effect sizes of subgroup analyses according to age, sex, measured skeletal site, type of SSBs, and SSBs intake questionnaire are summarized in Table 6. There was a large effect on whole body BMD (ES: -0.94, 95% CI: -1.54, -0.40). High consumption of SSBs had no effect on BMD at the heel, lumbar spine, total hip, mid-shaft radius, femoral neck, whole femur or distal radius. There was a moderate effect on BMD in females (ES: -0.50, 95% CI: -0.87, -0.13), but SSB consumption showed no association with BMD in males. There was a moderate or large effect on BMD in individuals aged under 30 years (ES: -0.57, 95% CI: -0.97, -0.17) and 30 to 50 years (ES: -1.33, 95% CI: -1.72, -0.93). Meanwhile, SSB consumption showed no association with BMD in participants older than 50 years of age (95% CI: -0.34, 0.17). High consumption of carbonated beverages had a moderate effect on BMD (ES: -0.73, 95% CI: -1.12, -0.35), but consumption of coffee with sugar showed no association with BMD. Articles using the modified FFQ and questionnaire developed by author found a large effect on BMD (modified FFQ: ES -0.96, 95% CI: -1.56, -0.37; questionnaire developed by author: ES -1.05, 95% CI: -1.68, -0.42)

Table 6. Sub-group analysis of associations between sugar-sweetened beverage consumption and bone mineral density in different age groups, sex, skeletal site, SSBs type, and SSBs intake questionnaire[1]

	No. of studies	No. of participants	ES	95% CI	I^2 (%)	p-value
Age						
< 30 years	7	3,122	-0.57	-0.97 to -0.17*	91	p<0.01
30–50 years	2	164	-1.33	-1.72 to -0.93*	0	-†
> 50 years	1	1,000	-0.13	-0.38 to 0.13	-†	p=0.40
Sex						
Male	3	1,382	-1.20	-2.75 to 0.36	96	p<0.01
Female	7	2,930	-0.50	-0.87 to -0.13*	88	p<0.01
Skeletal site						
Distal radius (g/cm²)	1	1,000	0.06	-0.19 to 0.32	-†	-†
Femoral neck	2	2,499	0.06	-0.11 to 0.24	53	p=0.14
Heel (g/cm²)	3	463	-0.38	-1.78 to 0.01	65	p=0.06
Lumbar spine (g/cm²)	3	3,499	0.00	-0.19 to 0.20	68	p=0.04
Mid-shaft radius (g/cm²)	1	1,000	0.00	-0.26 to 0.26	-†	-†
Total hip (g/cm²)	1	1,000	-0.19	-0.45 to 0.06	-†	-†
Whole body (g/cm²)	6	2,849	-0.97	-1.54 to -0.40*	94	p<0.01
Whole femur (g/cm²)	2	2,499	0.03	-0.09 to 0.15	0	p=0.40
SSBs types						
Carbonated beverages	9	4,179	-0.73	-1.12 to -0.35*	92	p<0.01
Coffee with sugar	1	133	-0.11	-0.50 to 0.27	-†	-†
Assessment method of SSBs						
Questionnaire developed by author	6	1,579	-1.05	-1.68 to -0.42*	92	p<0.01
24hr-dietary recall	3	2,632	0.03	-0.08 to 0.15	0	p=0.45
Modified FFQ	1	101	-0.96	-1.56 to -0.37*	-†	-†

[1]95% CI, 95% confidence interval; ES, effect size; I^2, FFQ, food-frequency questionnaires; I-square (%); p, p-value; SSBs, sugar-sweetened beverage. ES of 0.30 or less is regarded as small, 0.40 to 0.70 as medium, and 0.80 or above as large (24). *Effect size is significant with 95% CI. †Not applicable.

4. Discussion

In this systematic review and meta-analysis of 26 original articles, we identified an inverse association between consumption of SSBs and bone health. Meta-analysis of six studies revealed a significant inverse relationship between SSBs consumption and BMD in healthy adults. Eighteen of the 20 studies excluded from this meta-analysis supported its findings.

Sugar is thought to have negative effects on bone metabolism through increased loss of urinary calcium and imbalance in calcium homeostasis; thus the impact of excessive consumption of SSBs on bone health has become an area of intense research interest (11, 55). We found that overconsumption of SSBs has an inverse relation on bone health as assessed by BMC, BMD, and the incidence of bone fractures. Carbonated drink or sugary coffee investigated in the relevant studies included in this review have other three major factors that influence bone metabolism beside sugar; phosphate, acidity, and caffeine (12, 13, 14). Acids are added to beverages to provide a tart/tangy taste (56). High phosphoric acid content affects calcium metabolism negatively, which when combined with low dietary calcium intake, could increase the risk of development of bone diseases (56, 57). The low pH of carbonated drink such as cola (pH 1.8) can cause a sudden change in the gastric pH and thus interrupt calcium absorption, impairing bone health (56, 57). Caffeine is another potential risk factor, although its role in bone loss is controversial (58). Caffeinated beverage consumption, such as soda and sugary coffee, has been linked to reduced bone density and increased fracture rate (58). High-fructose corn syrup (HFCS), or glucose-fructose syrup, is the main sweetener used in sugar-sweetened beverages (59). Over-consumption of HFCS has been shown to be related to renal dysfunction and mineral imbalances, which could adversely affect bone health (60). In a recent review paper, it was reported that caffeine consumption negatively affects the growth plate cartilage and bone health, through the alteration of pro-inflammatory and anti-inflammatory cytokines (61). The main source of caffeine is soft drinks, coffee, tea, and chocolate. Another review paper showed that excessive dietary phosphorus intake have negative effects on bone metabolism (62). This paper emphasized that soft drinks, in particular cola, is associated with altered bone metabolism, low bone density, and fracture in human studies (62).

Dietary calcium is the most important dietary factor for bone metabolism and bone health, and milk is an excellent source of calcium due to its high calcium content and high rate of absorption by the body (29, 44). Apart from the direct effect of sugar itself, overconsumption of SSBs is strongly associated with reduced milk intake, resulting in lower bone mass and higher bone fracture risk through insufficient calcium intake (29, 44). Eleven of the 22 original articles included in this review investigated relationships between SSBs and milk and/or intake of other calcium-containing products (30, 33-36, 41, 42, 45-48). Of these, seven studies reported inverse correlations between SSBs and milk and/or calcium consumption (30, 33-36, 41, 47). This review enabled us to confirm the relationship between high SSBs consumption and insufficient intake of milk and calcium. Two intervention studies that replaced milk with SSBs (29, 44) reported a link between milk and SSBs consumption. According to a short-term intervention study (44), high intake of cola combined with a low-calcium diet over a 10-day period induced increased bone turnover compared to high intake of milk with a low-calcium diet. Thus, the trend towards replacement of milk with cola and other soft drinks, which results in a low calcium intake, may inversely affect bone health. Another intervention study performed over 16 weeks (29) reported that replacing habitual consumption of SSBs with milk had beneficial effects on height, despite no changes in bone mass. Because milk and calcium intake are important for bone health (29, 44), overconsumption of SSBs, accompanied by a reduction in milk intake, inversely affects bone health.

Women tend to have smaller bones and lower bone strength as well as younger onset of bone loss than men, and are therefore particularly susceptible to osteoporosis (61, 62). Subgroup analysis revealed that SSBs consumption had a significant inverse relation on BMD in women only. In addition, in four articles that investigated men and women separately, a significant inverse relationship between

SSBs consumption and BMD or BMC was reported for girls and women, but not boys and men (34-36, 45, 47). In two studies (51, 52) included in qualitative review, a positive association between SSB intake and bone fractures was confirmed in postmenopausal women. These findings suggest that excessive SSBs consumption is more detrimental to female bone health than male bone health.

Bone mass increases rapidly during childhood and adolescence, and up to 90 percent of peak bone mass accrues during this time (10). Adolescence is known to be a period of remarkably high intake of SSBs, which is accompanied by a decrease in calcium and milk intake, and diet quality is often low (10, 11, 64). We found that frequent consumption of SSBs in adolescence had a detrimental effect on bone health and was often associated with low calcium, milk, or protein consumption which play an important role in bone health. These eating habits may make it difficult to acquire adequate bone mass or achieve peak bone mass, thereby increasing the risk of age-related osteoporosis in the future as well as increasing the risk of bone fractures in children. According to a longitudinal study (29), children who had a habit of overconsuming SSBs had low calcium, milk, vitamin D, and protein intake despite the importance of these factors in bone health. In addition, evidence is accumulating that suggests that eating habits in childhood have a great effect on eating habits as an adult (65). Therefore, efforts to control children's excessive intake of SSBs and to encourage healthy eating habits are important for maintaining healthy bone health and improving quality of life later in life.

Bone fractures, which are indicators of bone health, are also linked to SSBs consumption (32, 34). Frequent intake of SSBs and failure to achieve bone mass can ultimately increase the risk of fracture (51, 53). In all eight stidies included in this review, a positive association between SSB intake and bone fractures was confirmed in children and adults. In seven studies (32, 49, 50, 51-54), high consumption of carbonated beverages increased the risk of bone fracture by 1.3- to 4.69-fold. The one study (33) reported two-fold higher SSBs intake in participants with bone fractures and three-fold higher SSBs intake in participants with recurrent bone fractures compared to their counterparts. Our review confirms that overconsuming SSBs not only affects bone health, but also overall quality of life through increased bone fracture. Policy targets, such as those discussed in this report and summarized below, are needed to reduce sugary drink consumption in children and adolescents and subsequently improve child health. The relevant studies included in the meta-analysis set the standard for SSB intake to 1~3 servings per day or 3 servings per week. In participants who consumed more or less than this amount, SSBs consumption and BMD showed a significantly inverse relationship. The 2020 strategic Plan from AHA recommends no more than 3~4serving(360 kcal) per week from SSBs (8). The results may suggest that observing this recommendation could help maintain bone health in addition to lowering the risk of obesity, diabetes and cardiovascular disease.

Many systematic reviews and meta-analyses related to SSBs consumption have been conducted (66, 67). However, the majority of these reviews have focused on prevention of unhealthy weight gain/obesity (4) and associated conditions, such as type 2 diabetes, dental caries, or dyslipidemia (66, 67). Meanwhile, there have been few reviews on bone health. This review provides useful information about the relationship between SSBs intake and bone health. This review is, to the best of our knowledge, the first systematic review and meta-analysis to evaluate the association between SSBs consumption and bone health in children and adults. Our findings indicate that SSBs consumption is inversely related to bone health in children and adults. According to the Centers for Disease Control and Prevention (CDC), SSBs consumption is higher among low-income families than high-income families (6, 68). Therefore, policies and efforts to lower SSBs intake may improve the health of low-income individuals. There has been much discussion about the effects of SSBs on obesity and diabetes, and based on these evidences, limits on the intake of SSBs have been established. However, the effect of SSB on bone health has been inadequately addressed. It takes a very long time to determine the effects of dietary consumption on bone health. Therefore, research on this topic is bound to be limited.

However, this topic is an area that must be studied for public health, and that this study will be the cornerstone.

However, some limitations of this review should be noted. First, most of the individual studies included in this review were cross-sectional observational studies. However, we were aware that the nature of this topic would limit inclusion of many other studies designs Second, BMD in the included studies was not adjusted for potential confounders (gender, age, height, weight, physical activity, smoking, and alcohol use, among others). We addressed this limitation by conducting quality assessment, which included an evaluation category, to account for whether adequate adjustments had been made for confounding factors. Third, only six original articles were included in the meta-analysis; therefore, we were not able to evaluate heterogeneity in sub-group analyses. However, most of the 16 studies that were not included in the meta-analysis but included in the qualitative systematic review showed similar observations to those of the meta-analysis, gave strong supporting evidence to the results of the meta-analysis. Fourth, studies included in this review used different methodology of food intake investigation such as food records, 24-hr dietary recall, FFQ, or dietary history. While all of which are proven to be valid as common methods in food intake survey research, the inconsistencies in the methods are inevitable in this kind of study. Fifth, it was difficult to analyze the publication bias, because the number of studies included in the analysis is small.

5. Conclusion

In conclusion, this meta-analysis showed a significant inverse association between consumption of SSBs and BMD. The results of the qualitative review supported the finding that SSBs intake were linked to bone health. There has been a worldwide effort to reduce excessive consumption of SSBs by approaches including nutrition education, campaigns, and putting policies in place. We have confirmed that these efforts not only prevent obesity, diabetes, and cardiovascular disease, but also have a beneficial effect on public bone health.

References

1. Miller C, Ettridge K, Wakefield M, Pettigrew S, Coveney J, Roder D, Durkin S, Wittert G, Martin J, Dono J: **Consumption of sugar-sweetened beverages, juice, artificially-sweetened soda and bottled water: An Australian population study.** *Nutrients* 2020, **12:**817.

2. Lee H, Kwon S, Yon M, Kim D, Lee J, Nam J, Park S, Yeon J, Lee S, Lee H: **Dietary total sugar intake of Koreans: based on the Korea National Health and Nutrition Examination Survey (KNHANES), 2008-2011.** *Journal of Nutrition and Health* 2014, **47:**268-276.

3. Park S, Xu F, Town M, Blanck HM: **Prevalence of sugar-sweetened beverage intake among adults—23 states and the District of Columbia, 2013.** *Morb Mortal Weekly Rep* 2016, **65:**169-174.

4. Malik VS, Pan A, Willett WC, Hu FB: **Sugar-sweetened beverages and weight gain in children and adults: a systematic review and meta-analysis.** *Am J Clin Nutr* 2013, **98:**1084-1102.

5. Vargas-Garcia EJ, Evans CE, Cade JE: **Impact of interventions to reduce sugar-sweetened beverage intake in children and adults: a protocol for a systematic review and meta-analysis.** *Systematic reviews* 2015, **4:**1-8.

6. Rosinger A, Herrick KA, Gahche JJ, Park S: **Sugar-sweetened beverage consumption among US youth, 2011-2014.** 2017,270;1-8 .

7. Blecher E, Liber AC, Drope JM, Nguyen B, Stoklosa M: **Global Trends in the Affordability of Sugar-Sweetened Beverages, 1990-2016.** *Prev Chronic Dis* 2017, **14:**E37.

8. Lloyd-Jones DM, Hong Y, Labarthe D, Mozaffarian D, Appel LJ, Van Horn L, Greenlund K, Daniels S, Nichol G, Tomaselli GF: **Defining and setting national goals for cardiovascular health promotion and disease reduction: the American Heart Association's strategic Impact Goal through 2020 and beyond.** *Circulation* 2010, **121:**586-613.

9. Rizzoli R, Abraham C, Brandi M: **Nutrition and bone health: turning knowledge and beliefs into healthy behaviour.** *Curr Med Res Opin* 2014, **30:**131-141.

10. Perez-Lopez F, Chedraui P, Cuadros-Lopez J: **Bone mass gain during puberty and adolescence: deconstructing gender characteristics.** *Curr Med Chem* 2010, **17:**453-466.

11. Tucker KL: **Dietary intake and bone status with aging.** *Curr Pharm Des* 2003, **9**:2687-2704.

12. Ogur R, Uysal B, Ogur T, Yaman H, Oztas E, Ozdemir A, Hasde M: **Evaluation of the effect of cola drinks on bone mineral density and associated factors.** *Basic & clinical pharmacology & toxicology* 2007, **100**:334-338.

13. Amato D, Maravilla A, Montoya C, Gaja O, Revilla C, Guerra R, Paniagua R: **Acute effects of soft drink intake on calcium and phosphate metabolism in immature and adult rats.** *Rev Invest Clin* 1998, **50**:185-189.

14. Birkhed D: **Sugar content, acidity and effect on plaque pH of fruit juices, fruit drinks, carbonated beverages and sport drinks.** *Caries Res* 1984, **18**:120-127.

15. Haque M, McKimm J, Sartelli M, Samad N, Haque SZ, Bakar MA: **A narrative review of the effects of sugar-sweetened beverages on human health: A key global health issue.** *Journal of Population Therapeutics and Clinical Pharmacology* 2020, **27**:e76-e103.

16. Movassagh EZ, Vatanparast H: **Current evidence on the association of dietary patterns and bone health: a scoping review.** *Advances in Nutrition* 2017, **8**:1-16.

17. Händel MN, Heitmann BL, Abrahamsen B: **Nutrient and food intakes in early life and risk of childhood fractures: a systematic review and meta-analysis.** *Am J Clin Nutr* 2015, **102**:1182-1195.

18. Dodwell ER, Latorre JG, Parisini E, Zwettler E, Chandra D, Mulpuri K, Snyder B: **NSAID exposure and risk of nonunion: a meta-analysis of case–control and cohort studies.** *Calcif Tissue Int* 2010, **87**:193-202.

19. Wells G, Shea B, O'Connell D, Peterson J, Welch V, Losos M, Tugwell P: **Newcastle-Ottawa quality assessment scale cohort studies.** *http://www.ohri.ca/programs/clinical_epidemiology/oxford.asp* 2014.

20. National Institutes of Health: **Study Quality Assessment Tools| National Heart, Lung, and Blood Institute (NHLBI).** *National Institutes of Health* 2019.

21. Hedges LV, Olkin I: *Statistical methods for meta-analysis*: Academic press; 2014.

22. Higgins JP, Thomas J, Chandler J, Cumpston M, Li T, Page MJ, Welch VA: *Cochrane handbook for systematic reviews of interventions.* : John Wiley & Sons; 2019.

23. Huedo-Medina TB, Sánchez-Meca J, Marín-Martínez F, Botella J: **Assessing heterogeneity in meta-analysis: Q statistic or I² index?** *Psychol Methods* 2006, **11**:193.

24. Higgins JP, Thompson SG: **Quantifying heterogeneity in a meta-analysis.** *Stat Med* 2002, **21**:1539-1558.

25. Cohen J: **A power primer.** 2003, 427-436.

26. Higgins JP, Thompson SG, Deeks JJ, Altman DG: **Measuring inconsistency in meta-analyses.** *BMJ* 2003, **327**:557-560.

27. Winzenberg T, Shaw K, Fryer J, Jones G: **Effects of calcium supplementation on bone density in healthy children: meta-analysis of randomised controlled trials.** *BMJ* 2006, **333**:775.

28. Malik VS, Popkin BM, Bray GA, Després J, Hu FB: **Sugar-sweetened beverages, obesity, type 2 diabetes mellitus, and cardiovascular disease risk.** *Circulation* 2010, **121**:1356-1364.

29. Albala C, Ebbeling CB, Cifuentes M, Lera L, Bustos N, Ludwig DS: **Effects of replacing the habitual consumption of sugar-sweetened beverages with milk in Chilean children.** *Am J Clin Nutr* 2008, **88**:605-611.

30. Fisher JO, Mitchell DC, Smiciklas-Wright H, Mannino ML, Birch LL: **Meeting calcium recommendations during middle childhood reflects mother-daughter beverage choices and predicts bone mineral status.** *Am J Clin Nutr* 2004, **79**:698-706.

31. Libuda L, Alexy U, Remer T, Stehle P, Schoenau E, Kersting M: **Association between long-term consumption of soft drinks and variables of bone modeling and remodeling in a sample of healthy German children and adolescents.** *Am J Clin Nutr* 2008, **88**:1670-1677.

32. Ma D, Jones G: **Soft drink and milk consumption, physical activity, bone mass, and upper limb fractures in children: a population-based case-control study.** *Calcif Tissue Int* 2004, **75**:286-291.

33. Manias K, McCabe D, Bishop N: **Fractures and recurrent fractures in children; varying effects of environmental factors as well as bone size and mass.** *Bone* 2006, **39**:652-657.

34. McGartland C, Robson P, Murray L, Cran G, Savage M, Watkins D, Rooney M, Boreham C: **Carbonated soft drink consumption and bone mineral density in adolescence: the Northern Ireland Young Hearts project.** *Journal of bone and mineral research* 2003, **18**:1563-1569.

35. Nassar M, Emam E, Shatla R, Fouad D, Zayed A, Atteya M: **Sugar sweetened beverages consumption in preadolescent children: 25-hydroxy vitamin D and bone mineral density affection.** *Journal of Advances in Medicine and Medical Research* 2014, 1400-1412.

36. Whiting SJ, Healey A, Psiuk S, Mirwald R, Kowalski K, Bailey DA: **Relationship between carbonated and other low nutrient dense beverages and bone mineral content of adolescents.** *Nutr Res* 2001, **21**:1107-1115.

37. Alghadir AH, Gabr SA, Al-Eisa E: **Physical activity and lifestyle effects on bone mineral density among young adults: sociodemographic and biochemical analysis.** *Journal of physical therapy science* 2015, **27**:2261-2270.

38. Cho DS, Lee JY: **Bone mineral density and factors affecting in female college students.** *Korean Journal of Women Health Nursing* 2008, **14**:297-305.

39. Hammad LF, Benajiba N: **Lifestyle factors influencing bone health in young adult women in Saudi Arabia.** *African health sciences* 2017, **17**:524-531.

40. Høstmark AT: **The Oslo Health Study: a Dietary Index estimating high intake of soft drinks and low intake of fruits and vegetables was positively associated with components of the metabolic syndrome.** *Applied Physiology, Nutrition, and Metabolism* 2010, **35**:816-825.

41. Jeong H, Yun S, Kim M: **Evaluation of food and nutrient intake by food frequency questionnaire between normal and risk groups according to the bone mineral density of female college students residing in Gangwon area.** *Korean Journal of Community Nutrition* 2010, **15**:429-444.

42. Kim SH, Morton DJ, Barrett-Connor EL: **Carbonated beverage consumption and bone mineral density among older women: the Rancho Bernardo Study.** *Am J Public Health* 1997, **87**:276-279.

43. Kim Y, Yoo J: **Associations between cola consumption and bone mineral density in Korean adolescents and young adults: a cross-sectional study using data from the Korea National Health and Nutrition Examination Survey, 2008–2011.** *Journal of Nutritional Science* 2020, **9:e56**.

44. Kristensen M, Jensen M, Kudsk J, Henriksen M, Mølgaard C: **Short-term effects on bone turnover of replacing milk with cola beverages: a 10-day interventional study in young men.** *Osteoporosis Int* 2005, **16:**1803-1808.

45. Pettinato AA, Loud KJ, Bristol SK, Feldman HA, Gordon CM: **Effects of nutrition, puberty, and gender on bone ultrasound measurements in adolescents and young adults.** *Journal of adolescent health* 2006, **39:**828-834.

46. Supplee JD, Duncan GE, Bruemmer B, Goldberg J, Wen Y, Henderson JA: **Soda intake and osteoporosis risk in postmenopausal American-Indian women.** *Public Health Nutr* 2011, **14:**1900-1906.

47. Tucker KL, Morita K, Qiao N, Hannan MT, Cupples LA, Kiel DP: **Colas, but not other carbonated beverages, are associated with low bone mineral density in older women: The Framingham Osteoporosis Study.** *Am J Clin Nutr* 2006, **84:**936-942.

48. Yeon J, Bae Y, Kim M, Jo H, Kim E, Lee J, Kim M: **Evaluation of nutrient intake and bone status of female college students according to the calorie consumption from coffee containing beverage.** *The Korean Journal of Food And Nutrition* 2009, **22:**430-442.

49. Chen L, Liu R, Zhao Y, Shi Z: **High consumption of soft drinks is associated with an increased risk of fracture: A 7-year follow-up study.** *Nutrients* 2020, **12:**530.

50. Delshad M, Beck KL, Conlon CA, Mugridge O, Kruger MC, Hurst PRv: **Fracture Risk Factors among Children Living in New Zealand.** *Multidisciplinary Digital Publishing Institute Proceedings* 2020, **37:**19.

51. Fung TT, Arasaratnam MH, Grodstein F, Katz JN, Rosner B, Willett WC, Feskanich D: **Soda consumption and risk of hip fractures in postmenopausal women in the Nurses' Health Study.** *Am J Clin Nutr* 2014, **100:**953-958.

52. Kremer PA, Laughlin GA, Shadyab AH, Crandall CJ, Masaki K, Orchard T, Snetselaar L, LaCroix AZ: **Association between soft drink consumption and**

osteoporotic fractures among postmenopausal women: the Women's Health Initiative. *Menopause* 2019, **26:**1234-1241.

53. Petridou E, Karpathios T, Dessypris N, Simou E, Trichopoulos D: **The role of dairy products and non alcoholic beverages in bone fractures among schoolage children.** *Scand J Soc Med* 1997, **25:**119-125.

54. Wyshak G: **Teenaged girls, carbonated beverage consumption, and bone fractures.** *Arch Pediatr Adolesc Med* 2000, **154:**610-613.

55. Johnson RK, Frary C: **Choose beverages and foods to moderate your intake of sugars: the 2000 dietary guidelines for Americans—what's all the fuss about?** *J Nutr* 2001, **131:**2766S-2771S.

56. Calvo MS, Tucker KL: **Is phosphorus intake that exceeds dietary requirements a risk factor in bone health?** *Ann N Y Acad Sci* 2013, **1301:**29-35.

57. Guarnotta V, Riela S, Massaro M, Bonventre S, Inviati A, Ciresi A, Pizzolanti G, Benvenga S, Giordano C: **The daily consumption of cola can determine hypocalcemia: a case report of postsurgical hypoparathyroidism-related hypocalcemia refractory to supplemental therapy with high doses of oral calcium.** *Frontiers in Endocrinology* 2017, **8:**7.

58. Rai N, Sandhu M, Sachdev V, Sharma R: **Evaluation of Remineralization Potential of Beverages modified with Casein Phosphopeptide-Amorphous Calcium Phosphate on Primary and Permanent Enamel: A Laser Profiler Study.** *Int J Clin Pediatr Dent* 2018, **11:**7-12.

59. Tsanzi E, Light HR, Tou JC: **The effect of feeding different sugar-sweetened beverages to growing female Sprague–Dawley rats on bone mass and strength.** *Bone* 2008, **42:**960-968.

60. Karalius VP, Shoham DA: **Dietary sugar and artificial sweetener intake and chronic kidney disease: a review.** *Advances in chronic kidney disease* 2013, **20:**157-164.

61. Alswat KA: **Gender Disparities in Osteoporosis.** *J Clin Med Res* 2017, **9:**382-387.

62. Seeman E: **Sexual dimorphism in skeletal size, density, and strength.** *The Journal of Clinical Endocrinology & Metabolism* 2001, **86:**4576-4584.

63. Adler RA: **Update on osteoporosis in men.** *Best Practice & Research Clinical Endocrinology & Metabolism* 2018, **32:**759-772.

64. Gibson S: **Sugar-sweetened soft drinks and obesity: a systematic review of the evidence from observational studies and interventions.** *Nutrition research reviews* 2008, **21:**134-147.

65. Collison KS, Zaidi MZ, Subhani SN, Al-Rubeaan K, Shoukri M, Al-Mohanna FA: **Sugar-sweetened carbonated beverage consumption correlates with BMI, waist circumference, and poor dietary choices in school children.** *BMC Public Health* 2010, **10:**234.

66. Greenwood D, Threapleton D, Evans C, Cleghorn C, Nykjaer C, Woodhead C, Burley V: **Association between sugar-sweetened and artificially sweetened soft drinks and type 2 diabetes: systematic review and dose–response meta-analysis of prospective studies.** *Br J Nutr* 2014, **112:**725-734.

67. Narain A, Kwok C, Mamas M: **Soft drinks and sweetened beverages and the risk of cardiovascular disease and mortality: a systematic review and meta-analysis.** *Int J Clin Pract* 2016, **70:**791-805.

68. Ogden CL, Kit BK, Carroll MD, Park S: *Consumption of sugar drinks in the United States, 2005-2008.* NCHS Data Brief. 2011;71:1-8.

Appendix A. Forest plot of association between sugar-sweetened beverage consumption and bone mineral density: subgroup analysis

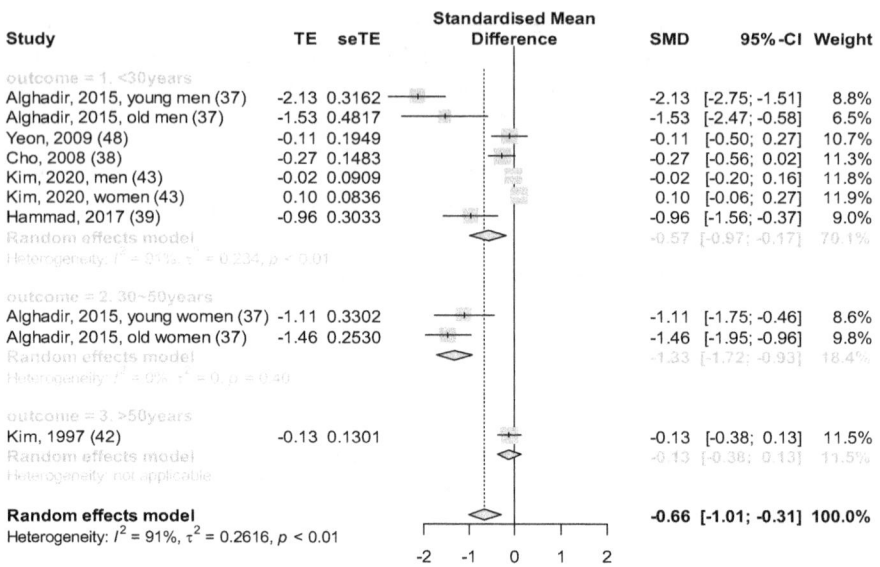

Figure A-1. Forest plot of association between sugar-sweetened beverage consumption and bone mineral density: subgroup analysis comparing by age

Statistical analyses were performed using the R program (mate-package, version 3.6.3). We conducted a meta-analysis according to a random-effects model (Hedge's method) for the main effect outcomes by combining inverse variance-weighted study-specific estimates. Squares and horizontal lines represent the effect size and 95% CI for individual studies, and the area of each square is proportional to the study's weight in the meta-analysis. Diamond and dashed vertical lines represent the overall effect size and 95% CI in the meta-analysis. The I^2 and P values for heterogeneity are shown. SMD, standardized mean difference; 95% CI, 95% confidence interval; W, weight.

(Continued)

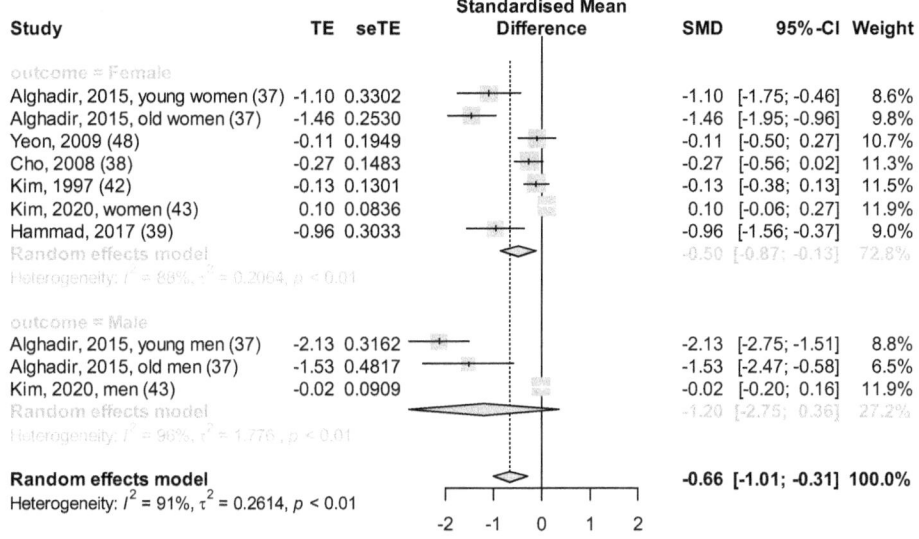

Figure A-2. Forest plot of association between sugar-sweetened beverage consumption and bone mineral density: subgroup analysis comparing by sex

Statistical analyses were performed using the R program (mate-package, version 3.6.3). We conducted a meta-analysis according to a random-effects model (Hedge's method) for the main effect outcomes by combining inverse variance-weighted study-specific estimates. Squares and horizontal lines represent the effect size and 95% CI for individual studies, and the area of each square is proportional to the study's weight in the meta-analysis. Diamond and dashed vertical lines represent the overall effect size and 95% CI in the meta-analysis. The I^2 and P values for heterogeneity are shown. SMD, standardized mean difference; 95% CI, 95% confidence interval; W, weight.

(*Continued*)

Appendix A. (*Continued*)

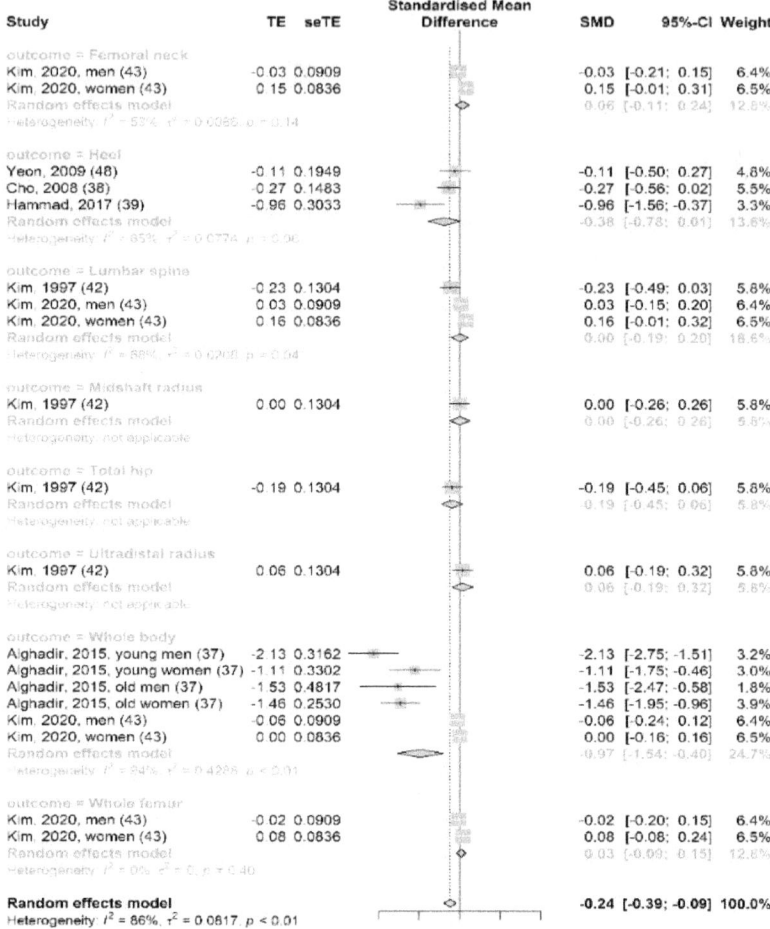

Figure A-3. Forest plot of association between sugar-sweetened beverage consumption and bone mineral density: subgroup analysis comparing by skeletal sites

Statistical analyses were performed using the R program (mate-package, version 3.6.3). We conducted a meta-analysis according to a random-effects model (Hedge's method) for the main effect outcomes by combining inverse variance-weighted study-specific estimates. Squares and horizontal lines represent the effect size and 95% CI for individual studies, and the area of each square is proportional to the study's weight in the meta-analysis. Diamond and dashed vertical lines represent the overall effect size and 95% CI in the meta-analysis. The I^2 and P values for heterogeneity are shown. SMD, standardized mean difference; 95% CI, 95% confidence interval; W, weight.

(*Continued*)

Appendix A. (*Continued*)

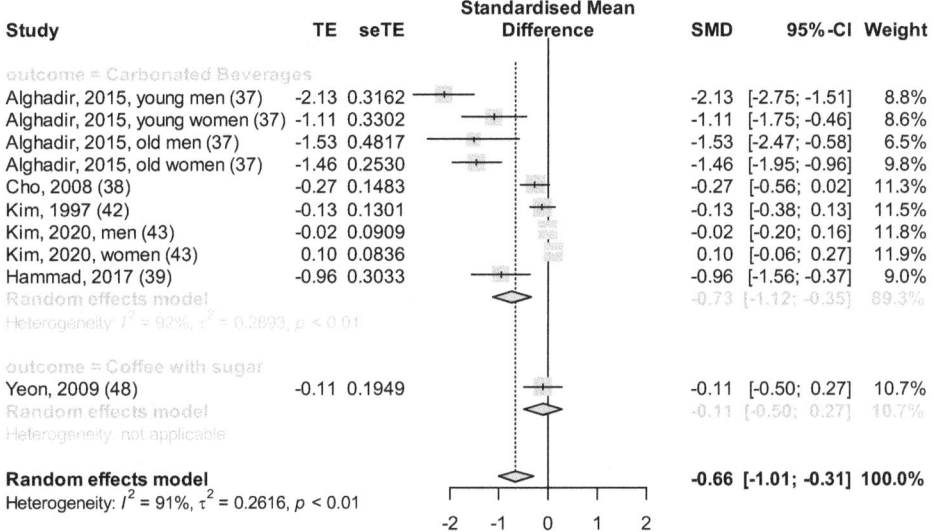

Figure A-4. Forest plot of association between sugar-sweetened beverage consumption and bone mineral density: subgroup analysis comparing by SSBs types

Statistical analyses were performed using the R program (mate-package, version 3.6.3). We conducted a meta-analysis according to a random-effects model (Hedge's method) for the main effect outcomes by combining inverse variance-weighted study-specific estimates. Squares and horizontal lines represent the effect size and 95% CI for individual studies, and the area of each square is proportional to the study's weight in the meta-analysis. Diamond and dashed vertical lines represent the overall effect size and 95% CI in the meta-analysis. The I^2 and P values for heterogeneity are shown. SMD, standardized mean difference; 95% CI, 95% confidence interval; W, weight.

(*Continued*)

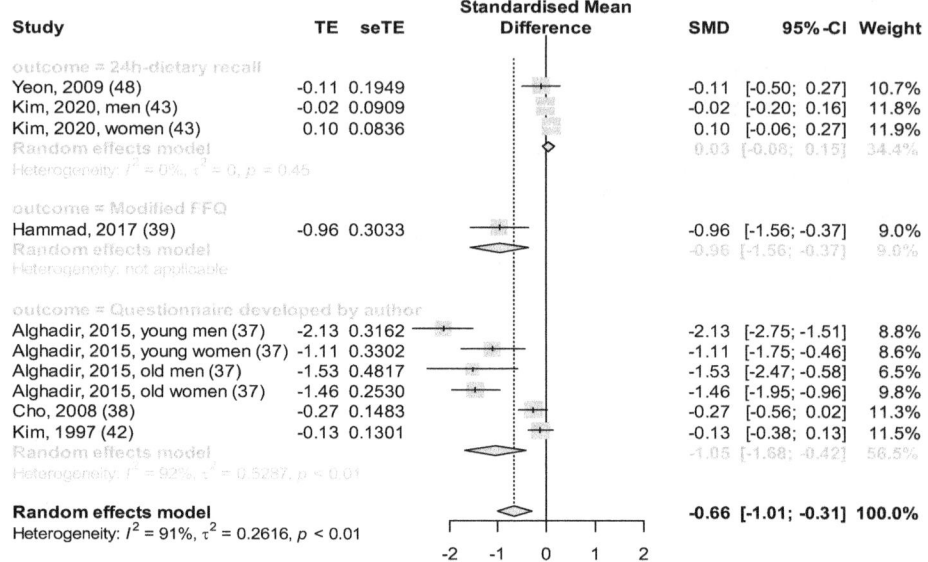

Figure A-5. Forest plot of association between sugar-sweetened beverage consumption and bone mineral density: subgroup analysis comparing by assessment method of SSBs

Statistical analyses were performed using the R program (mate-package, version 3.6.3). We conducted a meta-analysis according to a random-effects model (Hedge's method) for the main effect outcomes by combining inverse variance-weighted study-specific estimates. Squares and horizontal lines represent the effect size and 95% CI for individual studies, and the area of each square is proportional to the study's weight in the meta-analysis. Diamond and dashed vertical lines represent the overall effect size and 95% CI in the meta-analysis. The I^2 and P values for heterogeneity are shown. SMD, standardized mean difference; 95% CI, 95% confidence interval; W, weight.

Publisher: Eliva Press SRL

Email: info@elivapress.com

Eliva Press is an independent publishing house established for the publication and dissemination of academic works all over the world. Company provides high quality and professional service for all of our authors.

Our Services:
Free of charge, open-minded, eco-friendly, innovational.

-Free standard publishing services (manuscript review, step-by-step book preparation, publication, distribution, and marketing).
-No financial risk. The author is not obliged to pay any hidden fees for publication.
-Editors. Dedicated editors will assist step by step through the projects.
-Money paid to the author for every book sold. Up to 50% royalties guaranteed.
-ISBN (International Standard Book Number). We assign a unique ISBN to every Eliva Press book.
-Digital archive storage. Books will be available online for a long time. We don't need to have a stock of our titles. No unsold copies. Eliva Press uses environment friendly print on demand technology that limits the needs of publishing business. We care about environment and share these principles with our customers.
-Cover design. Cover art is designed by a professional designer.
-Worldwide distribution. We continue expanding our distribution channels to make sure that all readers have access to our books.

www.elivapress.com

www.ingramcontent.com/pod-product-compliance
Lightning Source LLC
Chambersburg PA
CBHW051251170526
45165CB00004B/1665